MW00425291

Dylan the Great Heart Warrior

Lived by Dylan

Author
Ty, Dylan's Mom

Illustrated by
Andrea Garcia and Ty

To Dylan,

You are God's Warrior

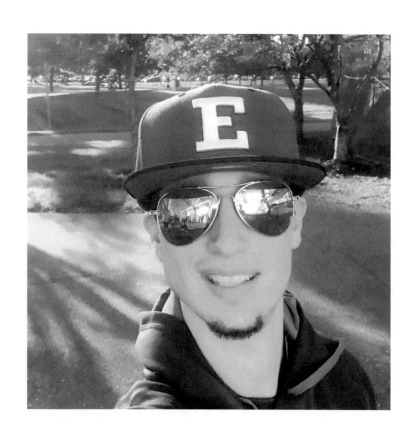

Dylan the Great Heart Warrior

All scriptures are from the Holy Bible, New International Version,
Grand Rapids, MI: Zondervan Publishing

Use of the University of Michigan trademarks (phrases, logos, and football uniform design in particular) is by the permission from the University of Michigan, Ann Arbor, Michigan.

Acknowledgements

Dr. Edward Bove MD, Pediatric Cardiac Surgeon
University of Michigan, C.S. Mott Children's Hospital

Dr. Albert Roccihni MD, Pediatric Cardiologist
University of Michigan, C.S. Mott Children's Hospital

Dr. Amnon Rosenthal MD, Pediatric Cardiologist
University of Michigan, C.S. Mott Children's Hospital

Ronald McDonald House Charities

Peter and Faye Renna
Printer's Press Inc. in Albuquerque, New Mexico

Patricia Woods, Editor

Robbie Kujath, Layout & Design

Preface

If you or someone you know is dealing with a congenital heart defect or any other serious medical issue, this book is for you! May it bring you hope and encouragement!

My son was born with a congenital heart defect. He was not expected to live through infancy, but he beat the odds! Now he is a young man attending Eastern Michigan University.

This book is true and the stories are real.

It is a book of God's promises for the one in 110 children born with a congenital heart defect, also known as CHD. Over 40,000 children are born each year with a congenital heart defect. There is no cure!

This is also the story of Dylan's life. As a young parent, I could not imagine the adventures we would have and the life we would live. Although very challenging at times, this journey has been one beyond our wildest dreams. Not one of us knows when we will be called home to our forever life in heaven, nor how the circumstances of life will alter our journey. I challenge you to live your life to the fullest every day. Find peace in the battle and joy in the storm. Do not waste your days in doubt or misery. Fight the fear, find happinesss and live the best life your situation allows. Be the hero of your own story. Let your life count!

You are the only you and that's your super power.

We hope "Dylan the Great Heart Warrior" inspires you to live!

This book is dedicated to Dylan, "The Great Heart Warrior", who is my inspiration in writing a book for all who walk the road you walk.

You are God's Warrior.

Introduction

When I was 22 years old, I gave birth to a full-term baby boy who was and is completely perfect. Immediately after his birth we knew there was something wrong. Dylan's skin turned blue and his oxygen levels were low. I had no idea what was about to unfold in his life. His condition got worse and we took him to Akron children's Hospital, where we found out that his heart was very, very, very sick. An echocardiogram revealed the severe level of Dylan's heart condition. His congenital heart defect is called Truncus Arteriosus, with an interrupted aortic arch, ASD, VSD, and discontinuous pulmonary right artery. He had only one kidney and some abnormalities with his left hand. The light of my little boy's bright future quickly grew dim.

He needed open heart surgery as soon as possible. I was devastated; I had never even heard of such a thing in an infant. I was told to find out what kind of insurance I had and to start praying. At that time, there were only three hospitals in the nation that could handle a heart like Dylan's. Boston Children's Medical Center, UCLA, and the University of Michigan C.S. Mott Children's Hospital.

Five days later we were on our way to Ann Arbor, Michigan for the first of five open heart surgeries to repair my son's very sick heart. Dr. Edward Bove is the cardiac surgeon who said they would find a way to repair Dylan's heart. This began our 24-year journey with CHD, Congenital Heart Defect.

Dylan's surgery was successful, but not without complications. The medical team experimented to find the best way to solve his problems. Some things worked, while others did not. Dylan's little body was so swollen after surgery that they could not close his chest for five days. His aortic arch repair caused many near-death episodes and at three months he had to have a second repair to add a one-inch graft to his arch. It was absolutely a mother's worst nightmare: I had to resuscitate him to prevent his death several times. Fortunately, the second repair was successful and his aortic arch has never caused him any more issues. But the memory of those fateful days cause me to reflect upon his early life experiences.

We spent four long months at C.S. Mott Children's Hospital, watching Dylan slip in and out of life. My three-year-old daughter Keysha was tossed around to families and friends who unselfishly loved and protected her. We lived at The Ronald McDonald House across the street from the hospital. It provided a haven for us. It was a place to rest, to eat, to get a shower and warm company. It was a place to run to during shift changes on the pediatric floors when we had to leave Dylan's room. It remains very near and dear to my heart as a wonderful, peaceful, and inexpensive place to stay. It holds priceless value to my family!

Dylan beat so many odds it is incredible. He was given a 20 percent chance to live. He suffered a traumatic brain injury that left his brain very small for his age. He developed a 65-degree scoliosis curve that was crushing his heart and lungs. He underwent an all-day surgery for that condition. The surgeon placed two 12-inch rods in his back with 18 screws. He lost almost all of his blood during the surgery and required a transfusion. He then had to have a diaphragm plication after a surgery left the diaphragm paralyzed up in his right lung. The new procedure allowed the lung to function again. Although his hand was webbed, it was the least of his worries. After several failed attempts to try to release the hand, we decided to leave it alone and concentrate on other things.

Dylan is a warrior. People who cruelly criticized him said he would never crawl, never walk, never talk, never have a normal childhood, let alone a normal life. We were told no contact sports, no contact play, and no rough-housing of any kind. The wrong bump on his chest could prove fatal. His life seemed more like a death sentence. The stories of each trial we encountered are endless. It was a rough time for the family and for a big sister who had to take on the responsibility of being the 'healthy one'. Many children in similar situations can relate to this title, and this is often as painful for them as being called the 'unhealthy one' is for other children. On the face of it, this life looked uninspiring. But, of course, that was not God's plan!

This book is about hope and encouragement for the actual inspiration that Dylan has been to all who meet him. An account of the beautiful life he has lived and the kind, caring, peaceful young man he has become. Through the tears and the pain, he has not only endured his birth defects, but he monumentally lives one great adventure to the next.

One might think the diagnosis of a congenital birth defect is a punishment, a form of a lesser life. It is an opportunity to see life as the fragile gift that it is.

Dylan has endured, suffered, hurt; but he has lived, laughed, loved and given his life all the effort and tenacity one young man can muster up. Through his faith he has overcome more obstacles than most would think humanly possible. He leaves the rest of us believing that he is a modern-day miracle. His life is a real testament to the power of God working in a life.

The adventures of "Dylan the Great Heart Warrior" are meant to breathe life and light into a family's very dark journey. It is meant to show you and your own heart warrior that no matter what happens, there is hope and that this life is yours to live. We encourage you to live it to the fullest no matter what might happen.

Dylan is now a young man attending Eastern Michigan University studying social work so he can eventually work with children who travel the same rough road he knows so well. He gives hope and encouragement using his experience and testimony to better a life with his great story.

He is "Dylan the Great Heart Warrior!" You're going to be one too!

"Praying activates the supernatural of God from Heaven; releasing God's Power, the Holy Spirit, and Heaven's angels to help us in our times of need."

-Pastor Galen Woodward
of Copper Pointe Church

I was chosen.
God authorized my life!

"My framework was not hidden from you when I was made in the secret place. When I was woven together in the depths of the earth, your eyes saw my unformed body. All the days ordained for me were written in your book before one of them came to be."
Psalm 139:15-16

"Before you were born, I set you apart."
Jeremiah 1:5

I am Dylan the great heart warrior!

I was sent to your universe by
my Mighty King and Savior!

Like all heart warriors, I was
born a world changer.

I live to have adventures even
when there's heart danger.

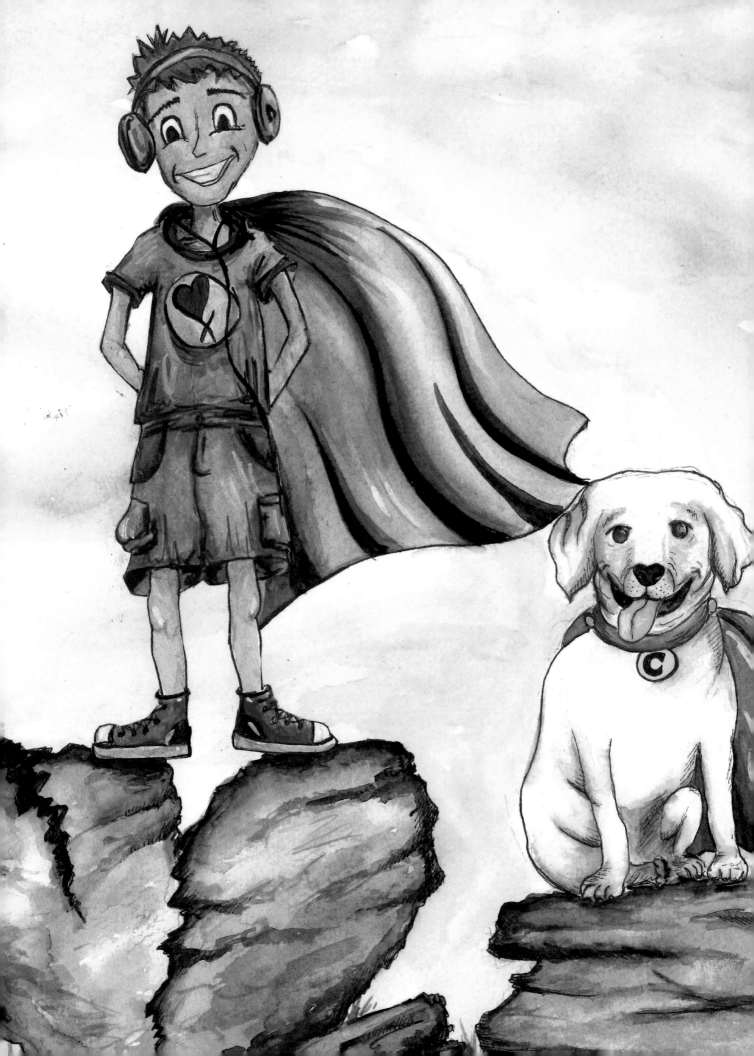

I came into this world a little different,
it's true!

I had trouble breathing, and
my skin was bright blue!

My journey is not of this world,
the things I go through.

The adventures of Dylan
are real and true!

"For God has not given us a spirit of fear, but of power and
of love and of sound mind!"
2 Timothy 2:7

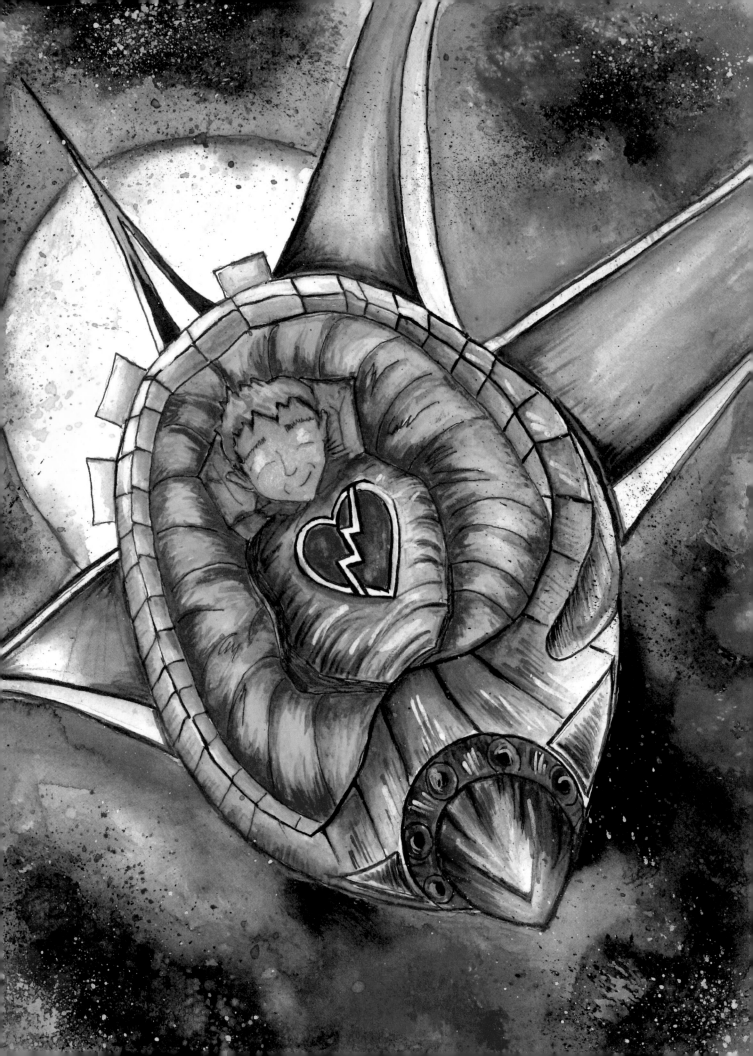

Like all great warriors
with a mission to do,

My journey started out
like bad voodoo!

My doctors geared up,
like a super hero crew,

Started my heart up like a
song I rock out to!

*"May the God of hope fill you will all joy and peace as you trust in Him, so that
you may overflow with hope by the power of the Holy Spirit."*
Romans 15:13

*"Say to those with fearful hearts, be strong do not fear;
Your God will come to save you."*
Isaiah 35:4

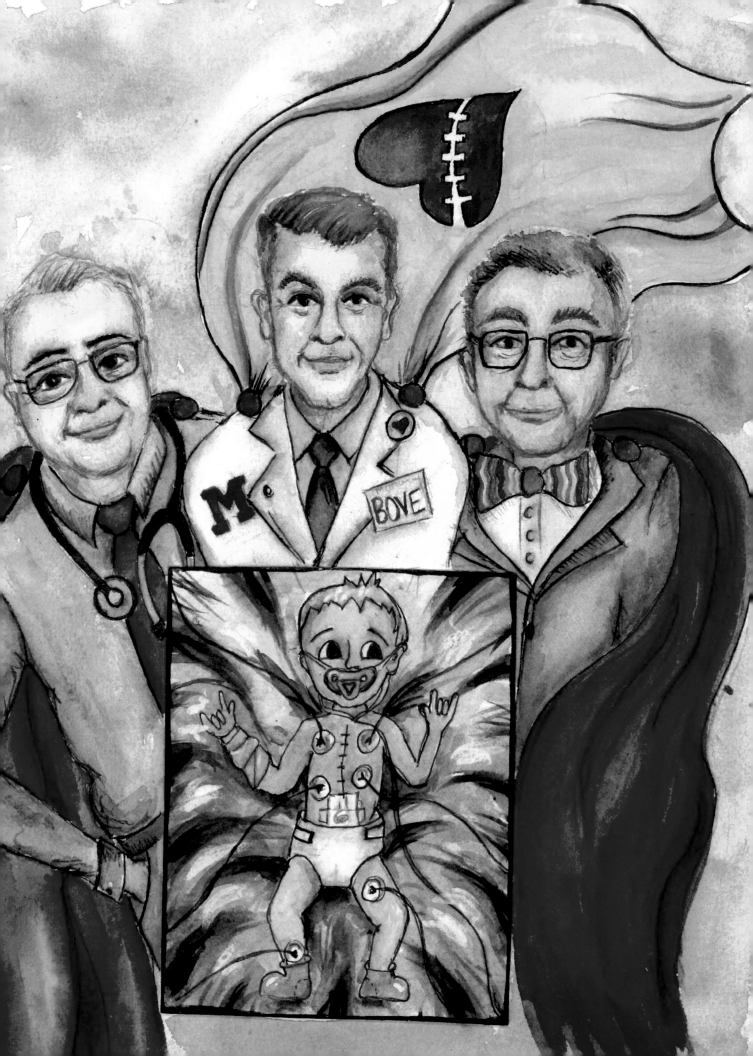

My heart wasn't pumpin',
but don't count me out.

Beating better than a drummer,
rippin' sick beats to wipeout!

One triumphant doctor said,
"I'll figure his heart out!"

Greater than a boxer with
a technical knock out!

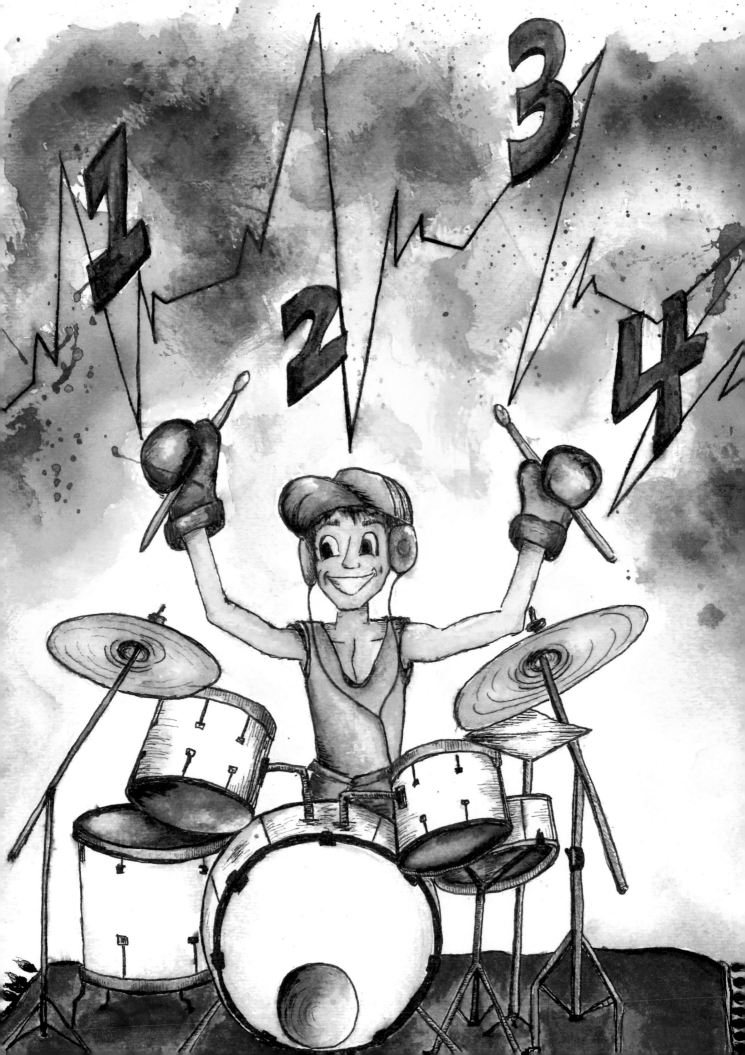

Modified hearts is
a medical specialty.

Mighty strength and courage,
with personal individuality.

You, too, will find out
life's possibilities.

Even ride supermotocross
like rad kamikazes!

"Be strong and courageous, do not be afraid or discouraged. For the Lord
your God will be with you wherever you go!"
Joshua 1:9

"And I am convinced that nothing can separate us form God's love. Neither
death nor life, neither angels or demons, neither the present nor the future, nor
any powers, neither height nor depth, nor anything else in all creation, will be
able to separate us from the love of God that is in Christ Jesus our Lord."
Romans 8:38-39

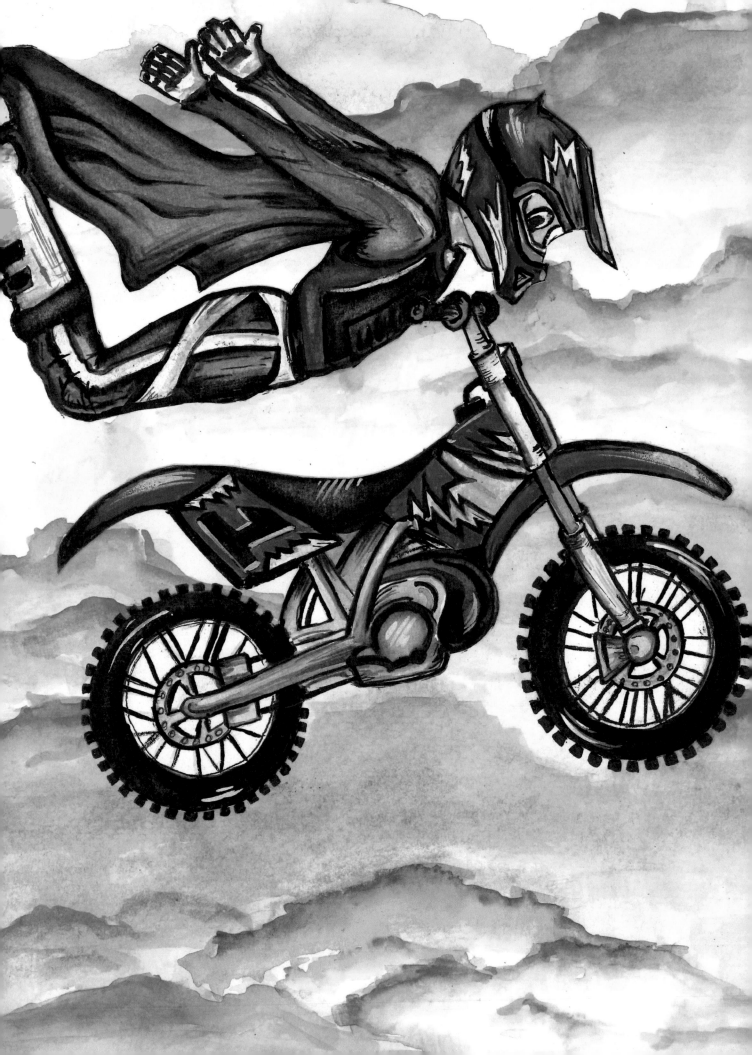

Some great heart warriors don't
think they're special at all.

Being so different feels like
a surfer on a beach ball!

Heart warrior rise up! Inspiration
born to be great!

Like America's birthday on the 4th
of July, you're a reason to celebrate.

"I sought the Lord and He answered me;
He delivered me from all of my fears."
Psalm 34:4

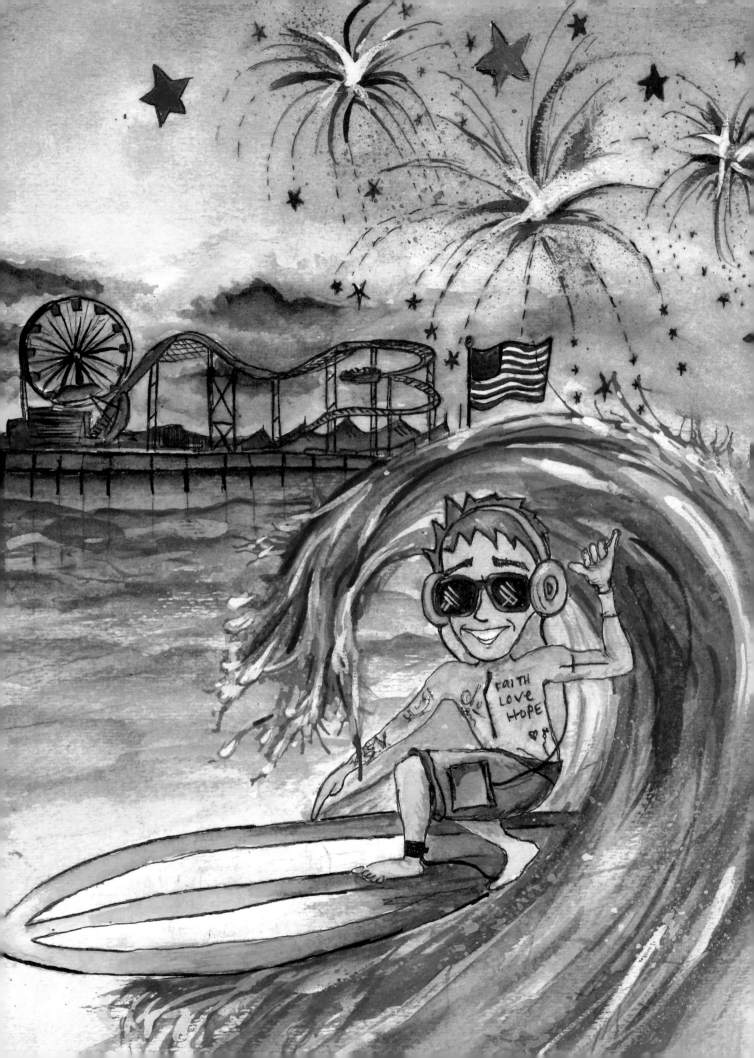

A prince to the King,
armed like a knight.

Or a brave soldier warrior
ready for a gunfight.

I have battled dark forces, like a superhero
fighting kryptonite

And I'm much more powerful
than a stick of dynamite!

*"Put on the full armor of God so that you can take your
stand against the devil's schemes."*
Ephesians 6:11

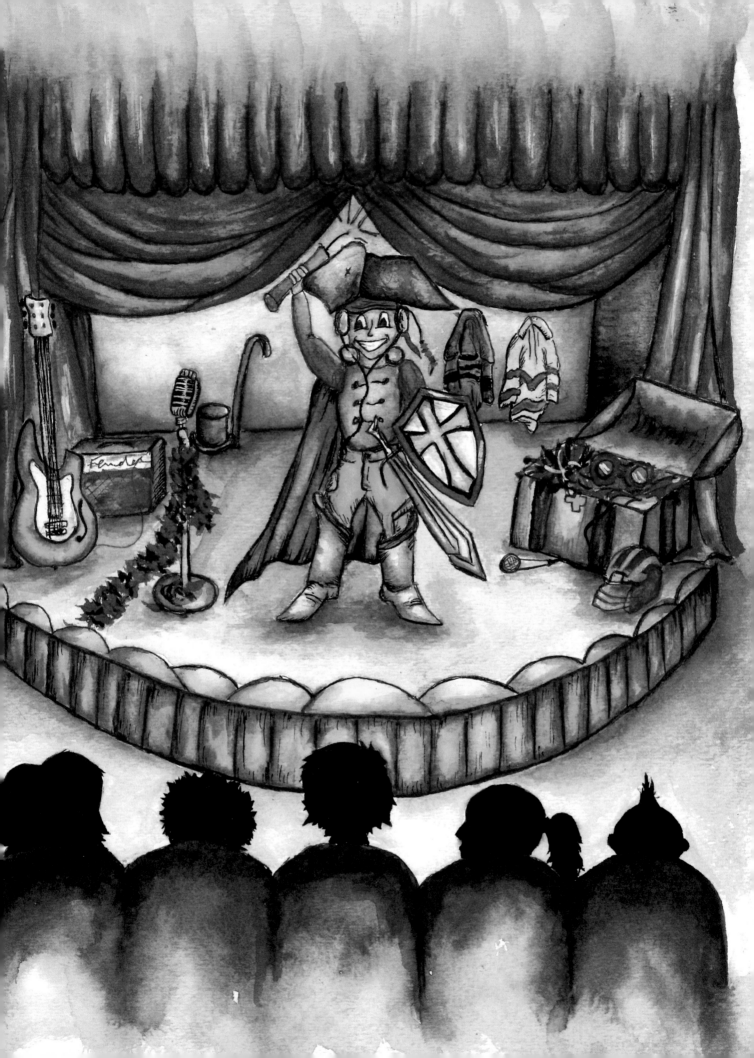

Heart warrior battles make
us nervous and sad.

Like a crazy bad crash,
you'll feel down and mad.

It won't last forever and
you did nothing wrong!

My music keeps me calm and
gives me strength for groovin' on.

*"The angel of the Lord encamps around those who fear Him
and He delivers them."*
Psalm 34:7

"When I am afraid, I will trust in you."
Psalm 56:3

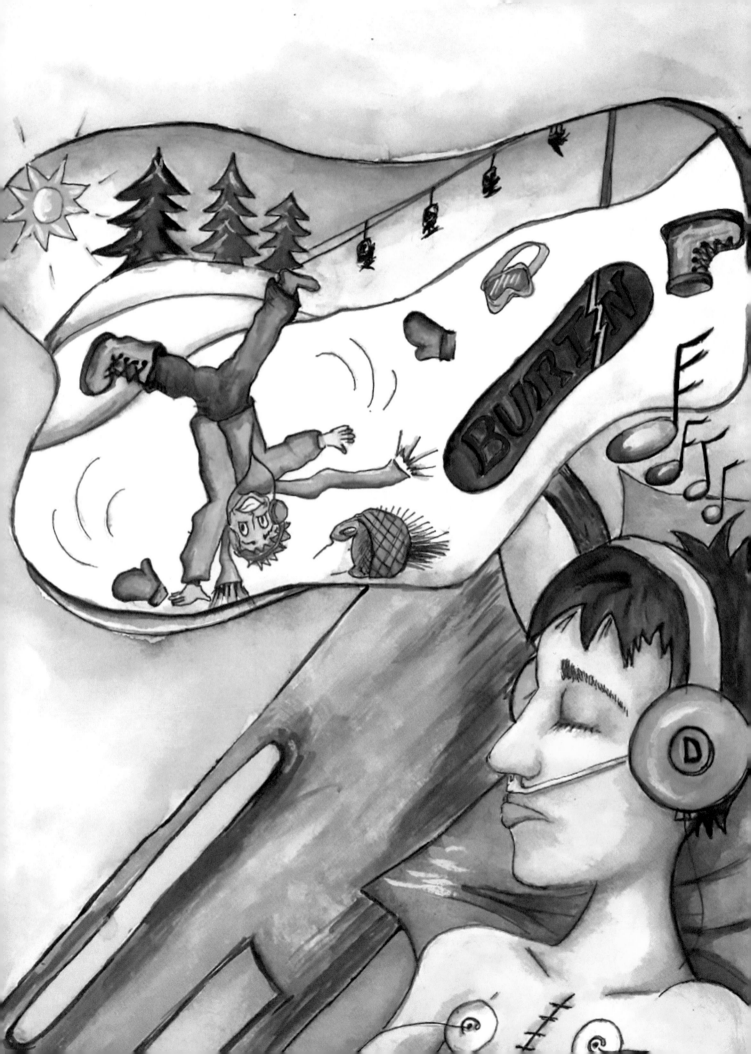

Like my favorite race-car driver,
I run my own race.

Even when it's hard,
I keep my own pace.

That's okay! I can do all things
with God's grace.

When the checkered flag drops,
I'm the winner in the showcase.

*"The Lord is my light and my salvation, whom shall I fear? The Lord
is the stronghold of my life of whom shall I be afraid?"*
Psalm 27:1

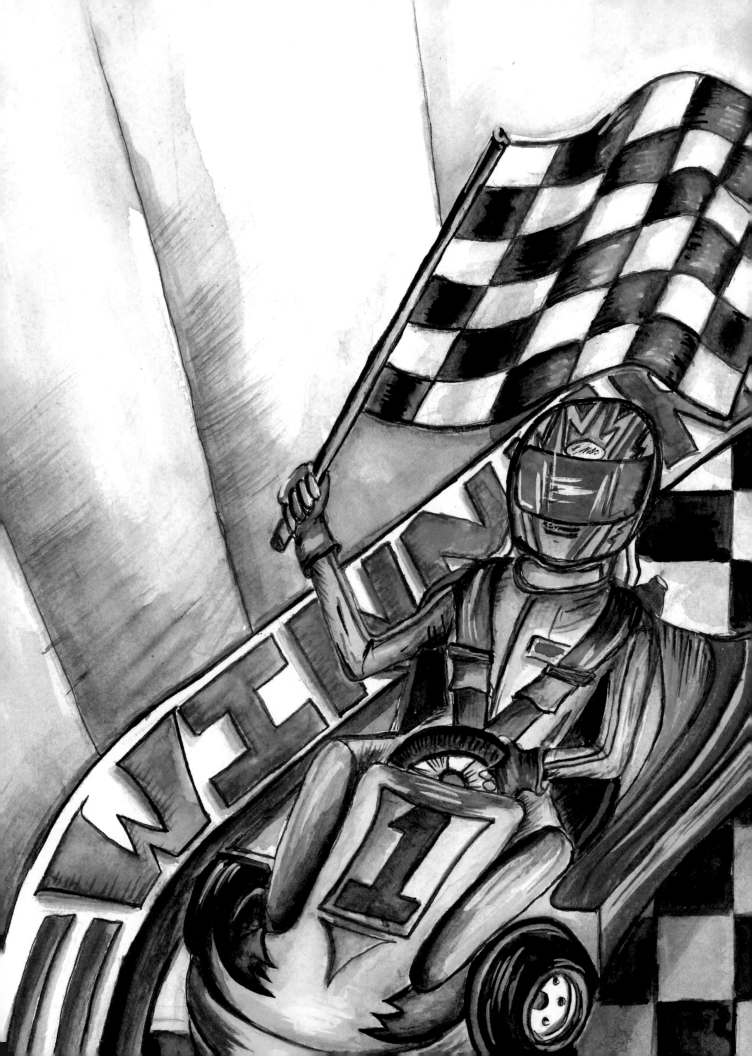

Greater than a football team that thinks they're really tough.

Having open-heart surgery can be really rough!

The scar is your trophy, and you are good enough!

"Hail to the Victors" of this congenital heart stuff!

"The angel of the Lord appeared to him and said, "Mighty Warrior, the Lord is with you!"
Judges 6:12

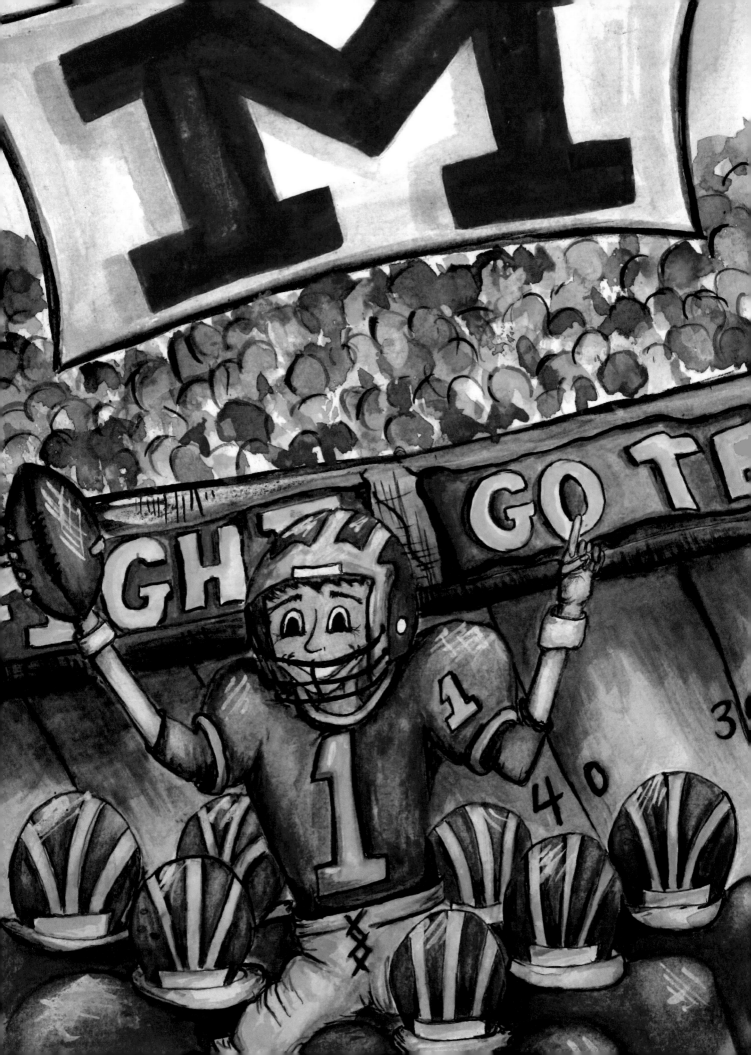

Hollywood movies need
a story like mine!

Love, action, drama,
better than Frankenstein!

I can be the director or
the hero made to shine!

In my dapper suit and tie, I'll take
the Oscar for my amazing story line!

"So do not fear, for I am with you; Do not be dismayed for I am your God.
I will strengthen you and help you; I will uphold you with my righteous right hand."
Isaiah 41:10

"God is our refuge and our strength,
an ever-present help in trouble."
Psalm 46:1

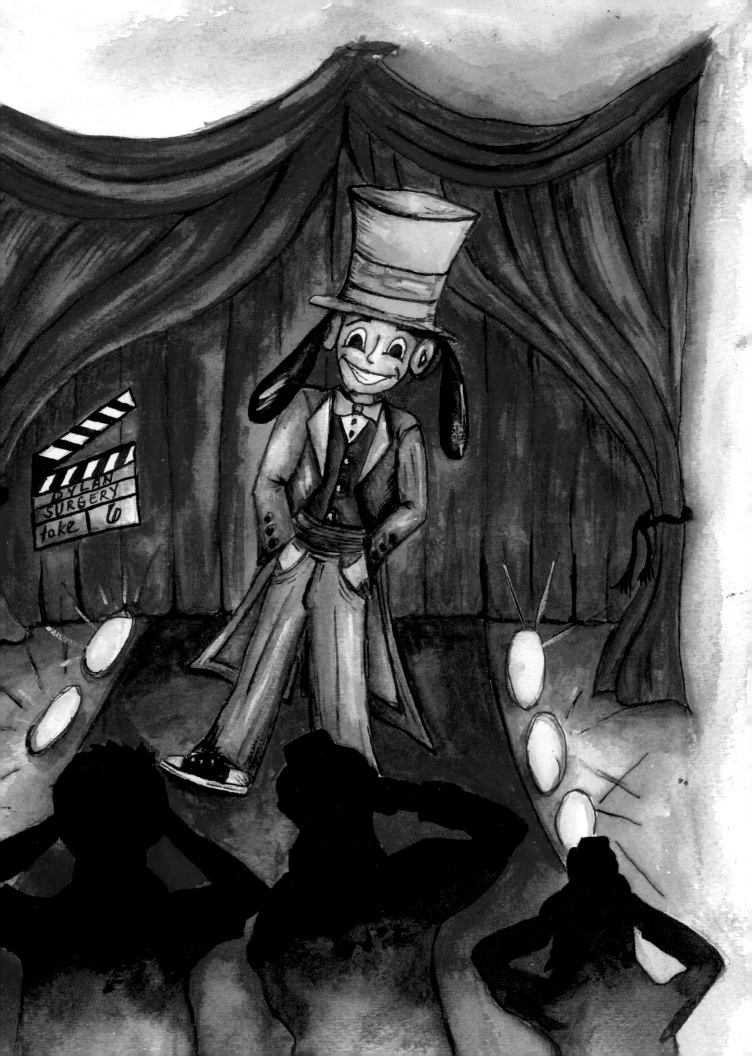

I have dreams that I'm living and
great adventures to come true!

There is nothing that can stop
what God wants to do!

Soar on wings like eagles!
A mighty mission for you!

I am the Great Heart Warrior,
you're going to be one too!

"Cast all your anxiety on him because he cares for you."
1 Peter 5:7

"He gives strength to the weary and increases the power of the weak.
Those who hope in the Lord will renew their strength. They will
soar on wings like eagles; they will run and not grow weary,
they will walk and not be faint."
Isaiah 40:31

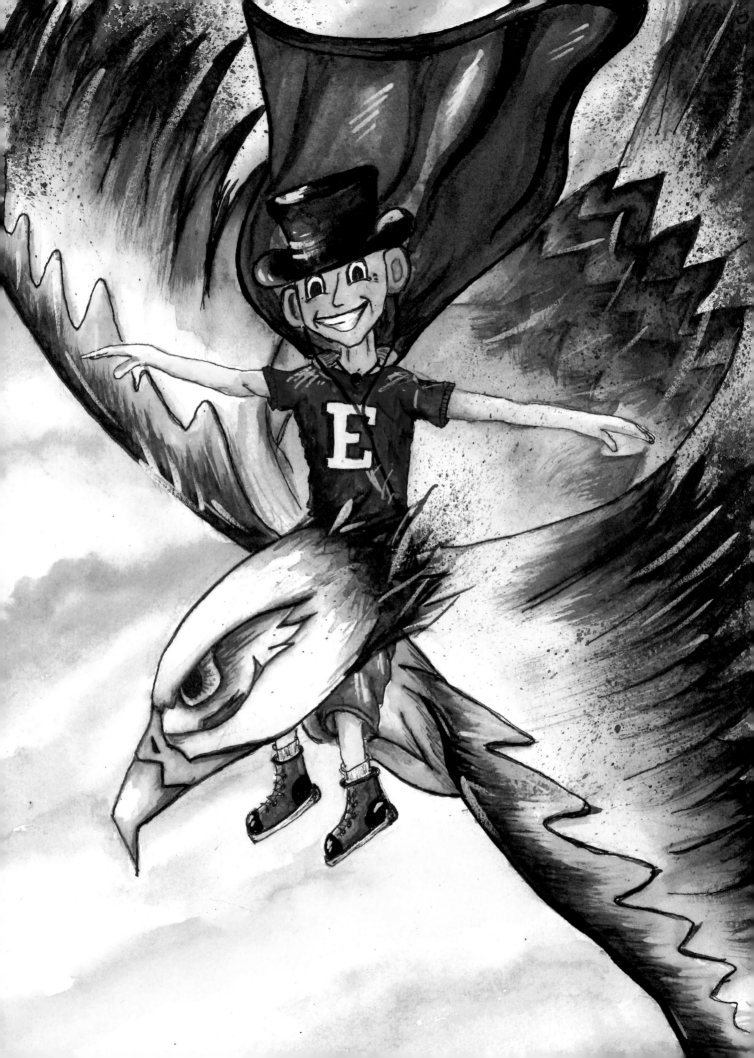

"Our Father in heaven,
Hallowed be thy Name.
Thy kingdom come,
Thy will be done,
On earth as it is in heaven.
Give us this day our daily bread.
And forgive us our trespasses,
as we forgive those
who trespass against us.
And lead us not into tempation,
But deliver us from evil.
For thine is the kingdom,
And the power, and the glory,
Forever and ever.
Amen."
Matthew 6:9-13

"The Lord is my shepherd;
I shall not want.
He maketh me to lie down in green pastures
and leadeth me beside still waters.
He restoreth my soul
and leadeth me in the paths of righteousness for
His names sake.
Yea, though I walk through the valley of the
shadow of death,
I shall fear no evil;
For Thou art with me;
Thy rod and Thy staff, they comfort me.
Thou preparest a table before me in the presence
of mine enemies;
Thou anointest my head with oil,
And my cup runneth over.
Surely goodness and mercy shall follow me all the
days of my life,
And I shall dwell in the house of the Lord forever."
Psalm 23

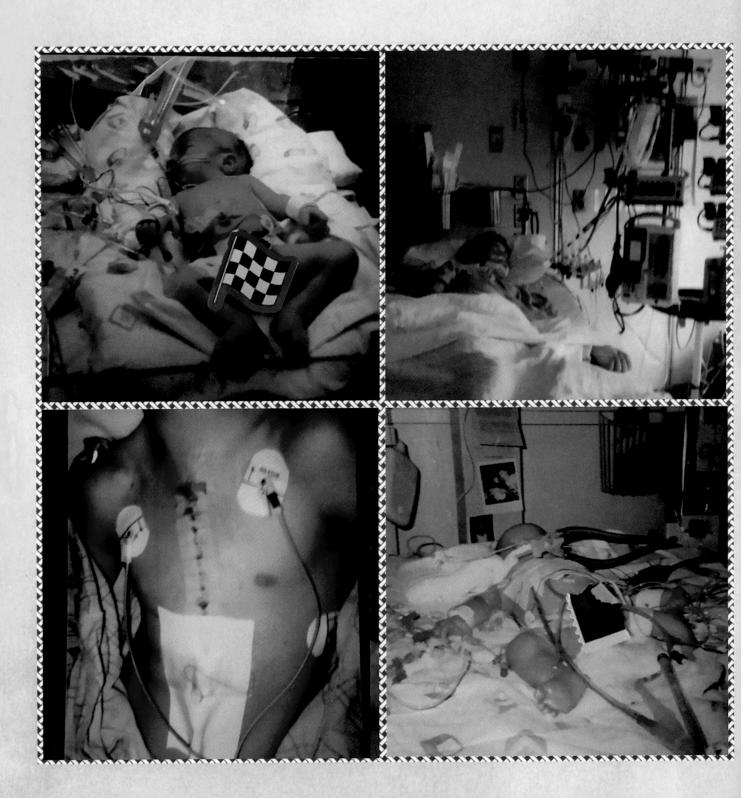

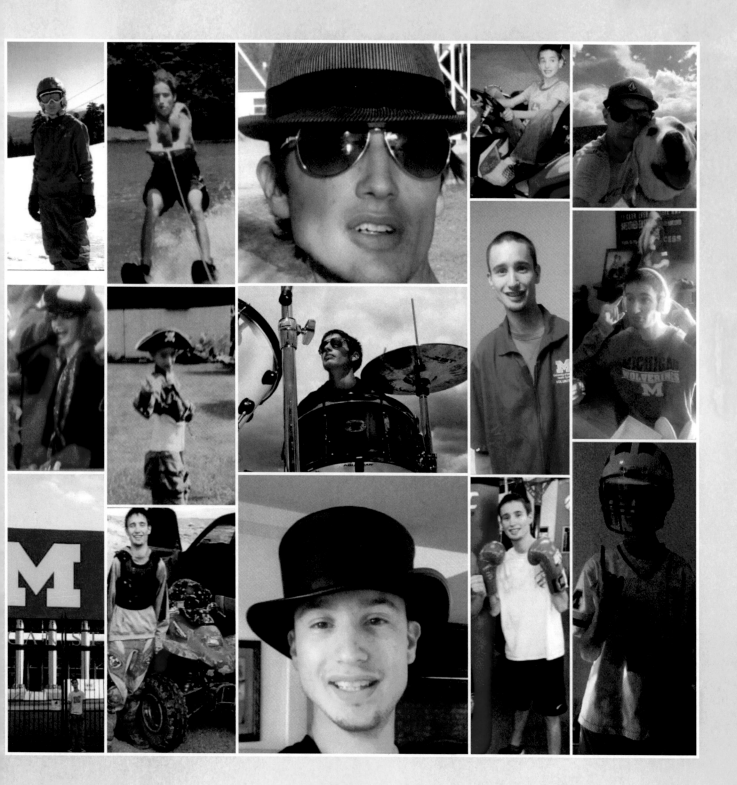

Psalm 91

Whoever dwells in the shelter of the Most High
    will rest in the shadow of the Almighty.
I will say of the Lord, "He is my refuge and my fortress,
    my God, in whom I trust."
Surely he will save you
    from the fowler's snare
    and from the deadly pestilence.
He will cover you with his feathers,
    and under his wings you will find refuge;
    his faithfulness will be your shield and rampart.
You will not fear the terror of night,
    nor the arrow that flies by day,
nor the pestilence that stalks in the darkness,
    nor the plague that destroys at midday.
A thousand may fall at your side,
    ten thousand at your right hand,
    but it will not come near you.

You will only observe with your eyes
and see the punishment of the wicked.
If you say, "The Lord is my refuge,"
and you make the Most High your dwelling,
no harm will overtake you,
no disaster will come near your tent.
For he will command his angels concerning you
to guard you in all your ways;
they will lift you up in their hands,
so that you will not strike your foot against a stone.
You will tread on the lion and the cobra;
you will trample the great lion and the serpent.
"Because he loves me," says the Lord, "I will rescue him;
I will protect him, for he acknowledges my name.
He will call on me, and I will answer him;
I will be with him in trouble,
I will deliver him and honor him.
With long life I will satisfy him
and show him my salvation."

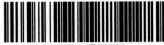

Made in the USA
Middletown, DE
01 March 2017